better nutrition *magazine* presen

GLUTEN FREE

by SHERRY TORKOS, BSc Phm

better nutrition
healthy living guide

Published by:
Active Interest Media, Inc.
300 N. Continental Blvd., Suite 650
El Segundo, CA 90245

This booklet is part of the *Better Nutrition Healthy Living Guide* series. For more information, visit www.betternutrition.com. Better Nutrition magazine is available at fine natural health stores throughout the United States. Design by Aline Design: Bellingham, Wash.

GLUTEN FREE

CONTENTS

better nutrition
healthy living guide

Introduction

My Personal Story

Good health is something that many of us take for granted. When I was young, I really didn't give my health a second thought. For the most part, I ate healthy meals, I had energy to play with my friends, and life was good. Years later as a teenager, I started to struggle with stomach problems. Initially my symptoms were minor and transient. Over time my problems worsened to the point that on a daily basis I suffered with stomach bloating, gas, pain, and diarrhea. As a shy teen, I was reluctant to talk about these issues with family and friends, but my symptoms soon become clearly apparent to others. I was losing weight, I suffered from extreme fatigue and headaches, my skin was pale, and I looked sickly.

My parents, eager to find out what was wrong with me, took me from doctor to doctor in search of a diagnosis. First I was told that I had irritable bowel, and I was put on a special diet. That didn't help. Then I was diagnosed with colitis and put on powerful sulfa drugs and prednisone. Again, this didn't help, and my situation started to deteriorate even more. The next doctor told my parents that he thought I was just an emotional teenager and that my issues were all in my head! Imagine that. I was physically ill with obvious symptoms. And despite my chronic diarrhea, I was instructed to increase my fiber intake and mix wheat bran into juice several times a day. At this point, I had lost more than 25 pounds, which was a lot for my 5-foot frame. I had diarrhea all day long, my skin was covered with eczema, I was anemic, my hair stopped growing, and I was emotionally depressed. These were all clear signs of malnutrition, yet somehow that was missed.

After much insistence by my parents, I was finally referred to a gastroenterologist. He was quite confident that the problem was not all in my head. In fact, during my first visit he told me that he suspected I had celiac disease, but properly diagnosing it would require a biopsy of my small bowel. This was the first time I had heard about celiac disease, so not knowing anything about it was a little scary. He told me that if I had celiac, it meant that my body was reacting to gluten, a protein found in many grains. And if the test was positive, I would have to give up many of my favorite foods such as pizza, breads, pasta, cookies, and other foods that contain flour. I recall thinking, "What is left?"

My biopsy ended up being positive. And while I was a little afraid of what life would be like as a celiac, I was relieved to finally, after many years of suffering, know what was wrong with me. It took me a while to adjust to the gluten-free diet since gluten is a hidden ingredient in so many foods. Eating out was dangerous. Despite my best efforts to explain my diet, I would end up getting "poisoned" quite often, and this would lead to a recurrence of my symptoms. When I was able to avoid gluten, my stomach symptoms resolved, but it took years for other aspects of my health to improve. My skin, hair, nails, energy levels, and even cognitive function were still not optimal. It was through my research and training in health and medicine that I discovered how to use supplements to correct the long-standing nutritional deficiencies that continued to affect my physical and emotional well-being. Now, 20 years later, great progress has been made in our understanding of celiac disease and its management. More and more restaurants and food companies offer gluten-free products, making it easier for those with celiac and gluten sensitivity. New supplements have been developed that help minimize the impact of hidden gluten in the diet, and researchers are continuing to explore ways to improve the lives of those with celiac.

In this booklet, you will find out about celiac disease and other conditions marked by gluten sensitivity; how to follow a gluten-free diet without feeling deprived; tips on dining out and cooking gluten-free; and how to use nutritional supplements to support your overall health.

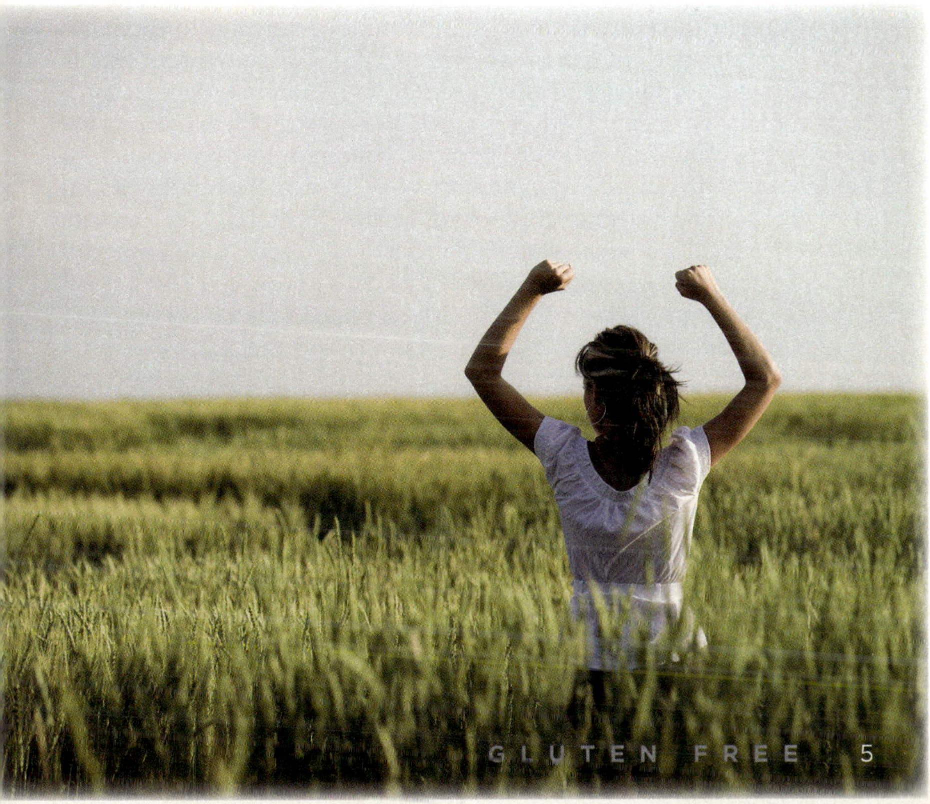

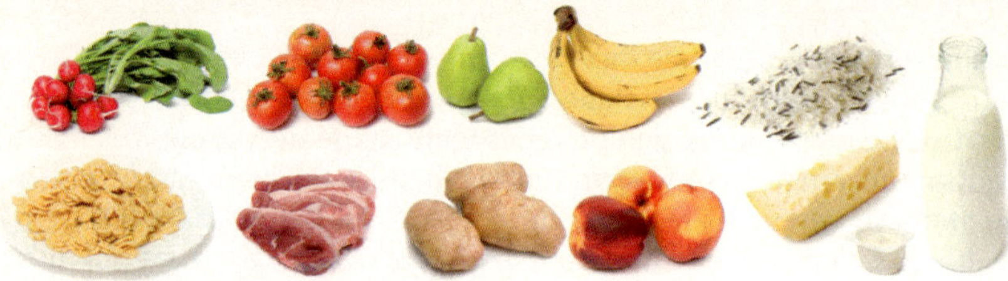

Chapter One

Celiac Disease And Gluten Sensitivity

Celiac (sometimes spelled coeliac) disease is also known as celiac sprue, nontropical sprue, and gluten-sensitive enteropathy. This disease is marked by an autoimmune reaction to gluten in the diet. Gluten refers to a group of proteins found in many grains such as wheat, rye, barley, triticale, spelt, and kamut.

In people with celiac, there is an autoimmune reaction to the ingestion of certain types of gluten. The specific types of gluten problematic for celiacs include gliadin in wheat, secalin in rye, and hordein in barley (oats contain a protein called avenin, which is also problematic for some celiacs). The damaging proteins are large molecules that are resistant to breakdown or digestion. In people with celiac disease, these proteins stimulate the immune system to produce antibodies. The antibodies attack the villi in the small intestine, which are fingerlike projections that make up the absorptive surface of the small intestine. This results in inflammation, damage, and destruction to the villi, which impairs the body's ability to absorb nutrients from food, leading to malnutrition and a variety of physical and emotional symptoms and serious health risks. In most cases, the damage is reversible when gluten is excluded from the diet.

The Gut And Beyond

When celiac disease was first described, it was thought that the disease primarily caused the classic gastrointestinal symptoms, such as bloating, abdominal pain, diarrhea, and constipation. Yet, according to recent reports, only 10 percent of those with celiac experience typical stomach complaints. It is now known that the disease can cause a wide range of both physical and emotional symptoms, making the diagnosis challenging. Some people with celiac disease may not have any symptoms. This is known as asymptomatic celiac disease. The undamaged part of their small intestine is able to absorb enough nutrients to prevent symptoms. However, people without symptoms are still at risk for the complications of celiac disease.

Some of the most common symptoms of celiac disease include:

- Gas and bloating
- Diarrhea or constipation
- Fatigue and weakness
- Headaches
- Weight loss
- Depression
- Irritability

In children, celiac may cause the child to have delayed development and growth, behavioral issues, difficulty concentrating, and poor memory.

Since celiac disease impairs nutrient absorption it can lead to malnutrition and symptoms of nutrient deficiency such as:

- Anemia and easy bruising
- Weight loss
- Delayed growth in children and short stature
- Infertility
- Peripheral neuropathy (nerve damage marked by tingling and numbness in the extremities)
- Dry skin and skin rash
- Joint and bone pain
- Muscle cramps
- Osteoporosis
- Discolored teeth
- Night blindness
- Irregular menstrual cycles
- Mouth sores or cracks in the corner of the mouth

Undiagnosed celiac disease increases the risk of developing other serious health problems.

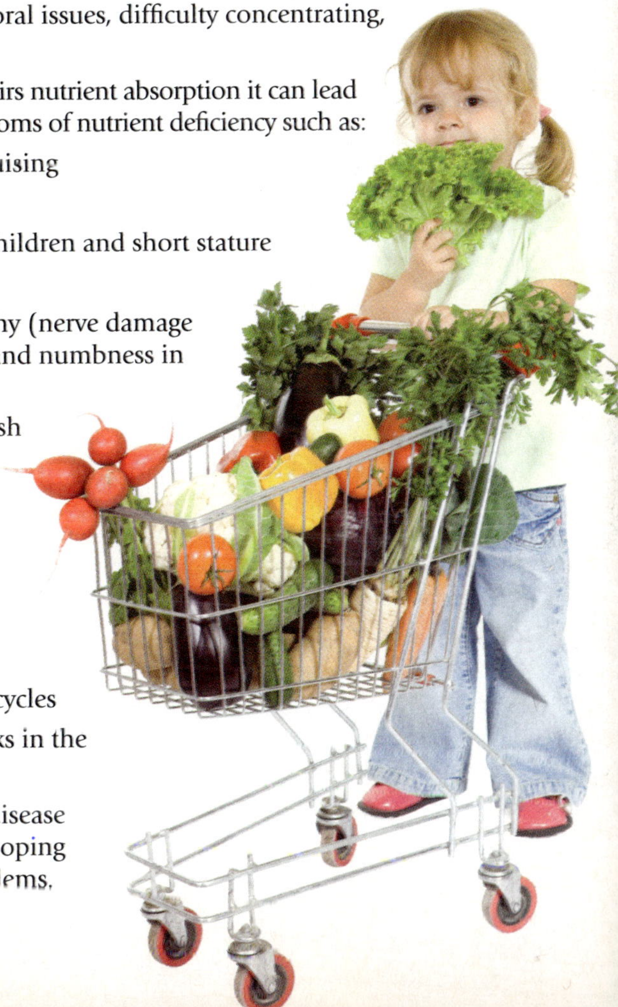

Cancer

Those with celiac are at increased risk of several types of cancer including: lymphoma, thyroid cancer, esophageal cancer, and cancer of the small intestine. In one recent report, it was found that celiac patients face a five-fold increase in the risk of developing non-Hodgkins lymphoma. While this is disheartening, the risk has gradually declined over the past few decades as the diagnosis and treatment for celiac has improved. In fact, in the 1960s, a population-based study reported that celiacs have a 100-fold increase in the risk of non-Hodgkins lymphoma compared to those without celiac.

Studies also have shown an increased mortality rate from cancer among celiac patients, meaning that they face a greater chance of dying from a cancer diagnosis. The risk of developing cancer seems to increase with delayed diagnosis and treatment of celiac. It is thought that the ingestion of gluten, which leads to continual damage to the intestine, an autoimmune response, and inflammation, are to blame.

It is important to realize that doctors now believe that following a gluten-free diet can reduce your risk of developing cancer to the same risk as that of the general population. In 1989, for instance, a medical study in Birmingham, England concluded that people with celiac disease who had followed a gluten-free diet for five years or more had the same risk of cancer as the general population.

Infertility

Infertility affects as many as one in six American couples during their reproductive years. Of those cases, about 15 percent result from no apparent cause. Recently, celiac disease has been identified as a significant, underlying contributing factor to female infertility. In fact, some research suggests that celiac disease is responsible for up to 8 percent of cases of unexplained infertility. Experts acknowledge that without treatment, celiac disease can cause repeated miscarriages and early menopause. Similarly, males with celiac disease often have gonadal dysfunction, which could also contribute to fertility complications.

Since celiac disease is an autoimmune disorder with a genetic component, a number of other autoimmune-mediated diseases have similar genetic linkages, such as type 1 diabetes, sarcoidosis, Sjogren's syndrome, thyroid disease, and myasthenia gravis. Studies have found a higher incidence of these diseases among those with celiac disease. Unfortunately, diagnosis and treatment for celiac disease does not cure these other conditions.

Related Food Allergies And Intolerances

Those with celiac may have other food allergies or intolerances. In particular, studies have found an association with both dairy and soy allergies. Those with untreated celiac may be at an even greater risk of having these other problems.

Lactose

Lactose is the naturally occurring sugar present in milk and dairy products. Many people with celiac develop lactose intolerance because gluten damages the intestinal cells that produce lactase. Lactase is the enzyme responsible for digesting lactose.

Lactose intolerance is actually quite common: It is estimated that up to 75 percent of the world's population is lactose intolerant to some extent. Symptoms of lactose intolerance include gas, bloating, diarrhea, and nausea. Not all people deficient in lactase have symptoms of lactose intolerance, but those who do are said to have lactose intolerance. In those with celiac, lactose digestion may improve once the intestines are healed.

Casein And Whey

With true milk allergies, people are allergic to either casein, whey, or both. Casein and whey are the two forms of protein in milk and milk products (e.g. cheese). Casein is found in the curd of the milk, and whey is in the liquid part that remains after the milk has curdled.

It is estimated that about 3 percent of the population is allergic to casein. Casein has a molecular structure that is quite similar to that of gluten, and like gluten intolerance, casein allergies are thought to be inherited. Symptoms of casein or whey allergies include hives, itchy skin, diarrhea, and respiratory problems (congestion). In extreme cases, milk allergies can be life-threatening.

Casein has been documented to break down to the peptide casomorphin, an opioid (morphine-like substance) suspected to aggravate the symptoms of autism. For those with casein or whey allergies, a dairy-free diet is recommended. Aside from milk and cheese, casein and whey may be present in hundreds of processed foods, such as energy bars, cereals, breads, and vegetarian meat substitutes. Casein may be listed as sodium caseinate, calcium caseinate, or milk protein.

Soy

Many with milk allergies turn to soy milk and soy products as a substitute. Unfortunately, a significant number of people with milk protein allergies develop soy protein intolerance when soy milk is substituted into the diet. It is thought that the intestinal mucosa damaged by cow's milk proteins may allow increased uptake of the potentially allergenic soy proteins. Allergic reactions to soy can cause rhinitis, rash and skin itching, asthma, diarrhea, gas, and in rare cases anaphylaxis, which can be fatal.

Soy protein intolerance is most common during infancy, and it usually regresses completely during the first two to three years of life. In a national survey of pediatric allergists, the prevalence rate of soy protein allergies was reported to be 1.1 percent, compared to the 3.4 percent prevalence rate of cow's milk protein allergy. The American Academy of Pediatrics recommends the use of extensively hydrolyzed or free amino acid–based formulae in the treatment of cow's milk protein allergy in infants and children. Most children can resume consumption of soy proteins by age 5. For those with continued reactions to soy, it means diligent dietary avoidance. Soy protein can be added to many foods such as energy bars, protein powder drinks, and packaged foods.

As with celiac, those with other suspected food allergies or intolerances should contact their doctor for proper testing and diagnosis.

Who Gets Celiac?

It was once thought that celiac disease was rare. However, with increased awareness and more accurate and accessible means for diagnosis, celiac has become a common condition. Approximately one in 100 to 133 people have celiac, yet only about 3 percent of these have been diagnosed. This means that 97 percent of cases are not diagnosed, leaving almost 3 million people in the United States alone at risk of developing complications from undiagnosed celiac disease.

Researchers have determined that celiac disease is a genetic condition, meaning that it is inherited and runs in families. Studies have shown that the familial occurrence of the disease ranges from 2.8 percent to 22 percent, depending on the study design and diagnostic criteria. The actual prevalence among family members may be even higher since many people go years without a diagnosis, and it is possible for people to have celiac without obvious symptoms that would lead them to get properly tested.

In a 2007 study published in *Digestion* researchers evaluated the prevalence of celiac disease in the asymptomatic siblings of celiac patients. It was found that an astonishing 23.8 percent (40 of the 168 asymptomatic siblings) were affected by celiac disease. Researchers concluded that silent celiac disease is 24 to 48 times more frequent in the siblings of celiac patients than in the general population.

Celiac affects both men and women, although more women are diagnosed than men—likely because women are more likely to seek answers and visit their doctor. The disorder is most common in Caucasians and those of European ancestry and very rare among those of Asian and Indian descent. It is believed that a person is born with the genetic predisposition to develop the disease, but it may not be activated for many years.

The Origin of Celiac Disease

Cereal grains have only been in the human diet for about 10,000 years—since the time of the agricultural revolution—which is a relatively short period of time in our evolutionary history. Researchers speculate that humans have not fully adapted to the digestion of the complex proteins present in gluten-containing grains. To make matters worse, our modern methods of growing and processing grains can make them even more difficult to digest.

Researchers have determined that celiac disease is a genetic condition, meaning that it is inherited and runs in families.

The first description of celiac disease goes back to the second century when Aretaeus of Cappadocia recorded a malabsorptive syndrome with chronic diarrhea. He referred to it as the "Coeliac Affection." The word coeliac originates from the Greek word for abdominal. Aretaeus believed that the problem was lack of heat in the stomach due to drinking too much cold water, which prevented proper food digestion.

In 1887, Samuel Gee, MD, gave the first modern-day description of celiac. He observed the symptoms of diarrhea, particularly in children, and suspected a dietary connection. Gee noticed that celiac children also had milk intolerance and recommended they avoid dairy and starchy foods (even rice, fruits, and vegetables) but, instead, consume raw meat and thin slices of toasted bread. While Gee was right about the dietary connection, he missed the mark with the offending food component.

The discovery of wheat as the culprit was made in the 1940s by a Dutch pediatrician, Dr Willem Dicke. His patients experienced improvement in symptoms during the Dutch famine of 1944, when flour was scarce. In 1952, a group of English doctors from Birmingham, England were the first to identify gluten as the offending component of wheat. They discovered damage to the lining of the intestine in those with celiac. In the years that followed, other symptoms and features of celiac disease were identified, yet there were still many misconceptions. Since celiac was most often noticed and diagnosed when the grains were introduced to the diet, it was thought that the disease primarily affected infants and young children. Many doctors who went to medical school in the 1950s and '60s were taught that celiac is a childhood disease. It was also thought (incorrectly) that celiac disease could be cured or go into remission and that a person could resume a regular, gluten-containing diet.

While it is not known exactly what activates the disease, three things are required for a person to develop celiac:

- **Genetic disposition:** being born with the genes linked to celiac disease, specifically the Human Leukocyte Antigen (HLA) genes DR3, DQ2, and DQ8
- **Trigger:** an environmental, emotional, or physical event, such as the introduction of grains to an infant's diet, adolescence, pregnancy, childbirth, infection, or undergoing a surgery, accident, or stressful situation
- **Diet:** eating foods that contain gluten, such as wheat, rye, and barley or their derivatives

Gluten Sensitivity And Other Health Conditions

Sensitivity to gluten has been associated with a variety of other health conditions including autism, attention deficit hyperactivity disorder (ADHD), schizophrenia, and dermatitis herpetiformis.

Autism

The possible connection between autism and the consumption of gluten (as well as casein—a protein found in milk) was first articulated in 1991 by a Norwegian doctor, Kalle Reichelt, who observed that people with autism had elevated urinary peptide levels. (Peptides are chains of amino acids.) Reichelt suggested that these peptides have an opiate effect on the brain, meaning they act like morphine. Other researchers supported this Opioid Excess Theory. It was hypothesized that incomplete digestion of gluten from grains and casein from milk leads to a buildup of peptides in the intestine, which cross into the bloodstream and enter the brain, exerting powerful effects on behavior and brain function. Studies proving or disproving this theory are lacking. However, many physicians advocate a gluten-free, casein-free diet for autism based on numerous case reports of beneficial effects for the patient. This type of diet is also recommended by the Autism Research Institute, a nonprofit group that funds research and provides information on autism and related disorders.

Facts About Celiac

Celiac is not simply a food allergy; it is an autoimmune reaction to gluten.

Celiac is not contagious; you cannot "catch" the disease. You may have it at birth but not develop an active form of the disease for many years.

There is no cure for celiac; dietary avoidance of gluten will keep the disease under control.

There is no "mild form" of celiac. You either have the disease or you don't.

Cheating on the diet, even if you don't develop symptoms, is dangerous because it can damage the intestines and increase your risk of serious complications.

Celiac affects both males and females, at any age.

ADHD

ADHD has also been associated with gluten sensitivity. Children with undiagnosed celiac could be misdiagnosed as having ADHD because the emotional and behavioral symptoms of celiac in children are similar to ADHD: behavior problems, poor attention, and learning delays. In a celiac, these symptoms result from poor nutrient absorption, and as noted above, gluten can have toxic effects on the brain.

ADHD is caused by a biochemical disorder within the brain itself that's thought to be associated with neurotransmitter deficiency. If a child's behavioral and/or learning problems are improved by a gluten-free diet, the child is not likely to have ADHD, but rather celiac disease. This is why it is so important that children with these behavioral symptoms be tested for possible celiac disease before a diagnosis of ADHD is made and any mood-altering medication such as Ritalin is prescribed, which could mask the true underlying cause. If the diagnosis of celiac is made and the child is put on a gluten-free diet, the gut will heal, digestion and nutrient absorption will improve, and in time this will have a positive impact on the child's behavior, learning, and development.

Schizophrenia

In the 1960s, Harvard researcher Curtis Dohan speculated that the low incidence of schizophrenia among those who lived in certain South Pacific Island areas was a result of a diet low in wheat- and milk-based foods. Dohan also observed the decreased incidence of schizophrenia in Germany during World War II when gluten-containing foods were scarce. He theorized that a genetic defect that impairs complete digestion of gluten and casein was a possible cause of schizophrenia. Dohan suspected that the incompletely digested gluten crossed into the bloodstream and disrupted brain chemistry, leading to the symptoms of schizophrenia. A clinical trial published by Dohan in 1966 suggested that a gluten-free diet could reduce symptoms in some patients with schizophrenia. Since then, several studies have examined the relationship between gluten and schizophrenia and failed to support Dohan's theory—until recently.

In 2004 researchers from Johns Hopkins University studied case records from 7,997 psychiatric patients in Denmark admitted between 1981 and 1998. They determined how many of these people had a diagnosis of celiac prior to being admitted for psychiatric evaluation. Taking into account other known risk factors, they found that the chances of developing schizophrenia were 3.2 times higher than expected in people with a history of celiac disease. Since many people with celiac go undiagnosed, the authors acknowledge that celiac disease was almost certainly underestimated in this study. Lead researcher William W. Eaton, PhD, says the next step is to determine if following a gluten-free diet makes a difference in the symptoms of schizophrenic people with celiac disease. He estimates that 3 percent of schizophrenic people could potentially benefit from such a diet.

Both schizophrenia and celiac disease involve a genetic component, and there is evidence of a genetic relationship between these two conditions. A variety of studies note a drastic reduction, if not full remission, of schizophrenic symptoms after gluten has been withdrawn from the diet. While larger studies are needed, the gluten-free, casein-free diet is safe and is often recommended by practitioners of functional and nutritional medicine for those with schizophrenia.

Dermatitis Herpetiformis

Dermatitis herpetiformis (DH) is an autoimmune disease associated with gluten sensitivity. It is marked by skin lesions (tiny blisters) with intense itching and burning sensations. These are located on the extensor surfaces of the elbows, knees, buttocks, and back. DH affects about 11 in 100,000 people, but in those with celiac disease, 15 to 25 percent are affected. It is more common in men and typically strikes in the second to fourth decade of life.

Like celiac, DH is associated with intestinal damage even though most people with DH have few or no stomach complaints or signs of malabsorption. Both DH and celiac patients not on a gluten-free diet have an increased risk of developing lymphoma of the small intestine, particularly when the condition has been present for many years.

The mainstays of treatment for DH are dapsone and a strict, gluten-free diet. Once DH is diagnosed and treatment begun, the response is dramatic, with the rash and skin burning resolving within days.

Chapter 2

Getting to The Grain

Celiac is considered the most common autoimmune disease, yet it is also highly undiagnosed. For many, the diagnosis of celiac disease comes after years of suffering, misdiagnosis, and frustration. According to a 2007 survey conducted by the Canadian Celiac Association, the average time to diagnosis is almost 12 years. The *American Journal of Gastroenterology* reports that in the U.S. the average is 11 years. Many people report having consulted with three or more doctors before their diagnosis was confirmed. I have personally met people who have suffered for longer than 20 years without knowing what was causing their symptoms. Health research experts estimate that some 97 percent of those affected by the disorder remain undiagnosed.

The diagnosis of celiac disease is challenging because of the wide range of symptoms and also because some of the symptoms mimic those of other conditions, such as Crohn's disease, colitis, diverticulosis, irritable bowel, and lactose intolerance. The latter is actually a common consequence of untreated celiac. There is also the common misconception that celiac is a disease of childhood, so some doctors don't think of it when they are treating an adult patient with gastrointestinal symptoms.

The diagnosis of celiac disease is made through a blood test and biopsy of the small intestine.

Blood tests for celiac disease, often referred to as the Celiac Blood Panel, measure:

- Total Immunoglobulin A (IgA)
- IgA antitissue transglutaminase (tTG)
- IgA anti-endomysial antibody immunofluorescence (EMA)
- If IgA is deficient, an IgG tTG test should also be ordered. At the discretion of the doctor, anti-gliadin IgG can also be ordered.

Researchers in Finland recently developed a home test for celiac disease called BioCard Celiac Test Kit. This test kit measures the presence of IgA in the blood with a simple finger prick, similar to checking blood sugar. In Canada, this kit is distributed by 2G Pharma Inc. and is sold in pharmacies, without a prescription, for $50. In the U.S., this test kit is currently being evaluated by the FDA and should be available soon. Greater access to an affordable and accurate method of testing for celiac will help facilitate diagnosis and treatment.

If the blood test is positive, then the next step is a small bowel biopsy. During this procedure, a tube is inserted down the throat, through the stomach, and into the end of the small intestine. An instrument removes tiny pieces of intestinal tissue, which are examined under a microscope.

In a person with celiac, the normal fingerlike projections (villi) are partially or totally damaged and flattened. The levels of enzymes located on the intestinal wall are also drastically reduced. One of these enzymes is lactase, the enzyme responsible for breaking down milk sugar (lactose) so it can be absorbed. As discussed earlier, intestinal damage and reduced lactase levels in an untreated celiac patient cause lactose intolerance. Elevated numbers of T-cell lymphocytes (white blood cells) are also present.

The diagnosis of celiac disease is complete when the person's health improves following implementation of the gluten-free (GF) diet. When gluten is removed from the diet, most of the damage done to the small intestine (the jejunum) is eventually repaired. It takes only three to six days for the intestinal lining (the mucosa) to show improvement. Within three to six months, most symptoms subside as the mucosa returns to its normal (or nearly normal) state.

If, after several months on the GF diet, symptoms persist, then it is important for the person to evaluate whether all sources of gluten have been removed from the diet. Even minimal amounts of gluten (bread crumbs in salad or fries cooked in oil with breaded items) can damage the intestine.

Note: It is important to continue eating a normal, gluten-containing diet before being tested for celiac. Having either the blood tests or a biopsy done after starting a gluten-free diet can give a false-negative result.

Genetic Testing

Celiac disease has a hereditary basis and is linked to genetically transmitted antigens known as histocompatibility cell antigens (HLA). Specifically they are HLA DR3-DQ2, DR5/7 DQ2, and DR4-DQ8. Genetic tests for celiac disease and gluten sensitivity are readily available. Testing can be performed on either blood or mouth-swab samples.

Depending on the laboratory, the tests can predict not only your risk of celiac disease but also the likelihood of your children inheriting the condition, your likelihood of more severe celiac disease symptoms, whether one or both of your parents had the risk gene, and even, at some laboratories, your risk of gluten sensitivity without celiac disease.

Chapter 3
The Gluten-Free Diet

There is currently no cure for celiac disease. Strict dietary avoidance of gluten is critical for the management and the prevention of complications. The good news is that about 70 percent of people with celiac disease respond positively to a gluten-free diet within days or weeks.

It is important for a newly diagnosed person to meet with a dietitian to find out about the gluten-free diet and all the possible hidden sources of gluten. Joining your local celiac association is also a great way to learn about gluten-free food products and restaurants that cater to celiacs. The Celiac Sprue Association of the United States and the Canadian Celiac Association are other great sources of information on the diet. These associations are also a great way to share your experience and to learn and help others. In the back of this booklet, I have listed books, Web sites, and other resources.

Common sources of gluten include:

- **Wheat and all its forms** including wheat starch, wheat bran, wheat germ, cracked wheat, hydrolyzed wheat protein, graham flour, durum, semolina, spelt, couscous, kamut, einkorn, and faro
- **Rye**
- **Barley**
- **Triticale** (a cross between wheat and rye)
- **Oats** (commercial forms)

Plenty of foods are naturally gluten-free, such as fruits, vegetables, eggs, dairy, nuts, seeds, beans, legumes, potatoes, corn, rice, and meats. Wine is safe. Many alcoholic beverages are distilled and, therefore, safe because the protein components are removed. Brandy, vodka, rum, whiskey, gin, and sherry are all gluten-free. Most beers contain barley malt; however, a few gluten-free beers are available that are made from rice.

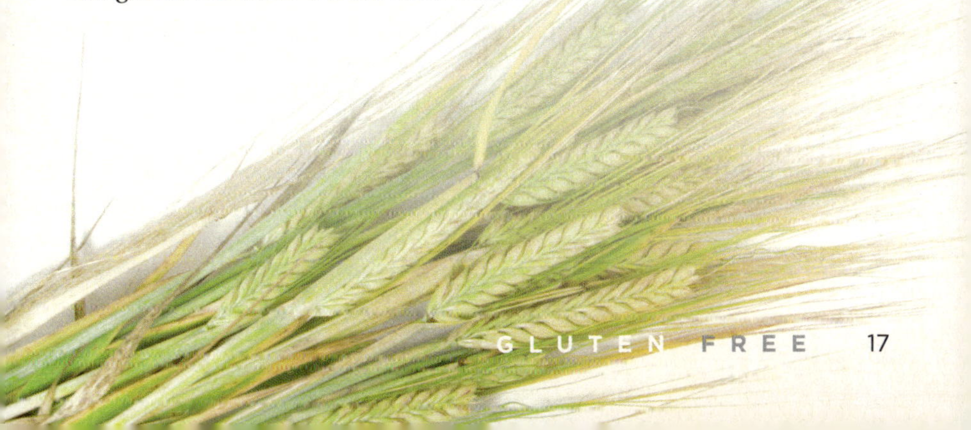

Here is a list of some other foods and grains that are gluten-free:

- **Amaranth**
- **Arrowroot**
- **Buckwheat**
- **Cassava**
- **Millet**
- **Oats** (pure; uncontaminated)
- **Quinoa**
- **Sorghum**
- **Soy**
- **Tapioca**

Many health food stores and some grocery stores carry the above grains, and flours made from these grains can be substituted in recipes.

To ensure that your body is getting a range of vitamins, minerals, and plant compounds, eat a variety of fruits, vegetables, and gluten-free grains. While many of us have our favorite foods, it is important to branch out and try new foods, so you can have the broad range of nutrients found in nature. Experiment with new foods and recipes.

The Oats Controversy

The safety of oats in a gluten-free diet is a controversial matter. Oats do not naturally contain gluten. However, like other grains, they can become contaminated during harvesting, transporting, milling, and processing. In the case of oats, the contamination can occur with wheat, rye, or barley, which is a problem for those with celiac disease.

A handful of studies suggest that pure, uncontaminated oats may be tolerated by some people with celiac disease. The problem is that these studies were done with small groups of people over short periods of time. Other studies indicate that some people with celiac have an immune response to oats, whether they are pure or not.

Currently, there is no way to identify which people with celiac disease may tolerate oats. Therefore, the Celiac Sprue Association of the United States recommends caution when considering the use of uncontaminated oats in a gluten-free diet.

Health Canada and the Canadian Celiac Association take the position that the majority of people with celiac disease can tolerate moderate amounts of pure oats. When people are introducing pure oats into their gluten-free diet, the associations recommend that individuals have proper follow-up by a health professional, including initial and long-term assessments. The amounts of pure oats should be limited to 20 to 25 grams per day (65 ml or ¼ cup dry rolled oats) for children and 50 to 70 grams per day (125 to 175 ml or ½ to ¾ cup dry rolled oats) for adults.

Those who decide to add oats to the gluten-free diet should have antibody testing and symptom screening by the physician. Pure, uncontaminated oats are available from a limited number of food suppliers including Bob's Red Mill Gluten-Free Oats.

Hidden Gluten

Gluten is in obvious places like breads, pastas, cookies, and other baked goods, but it can also be found as an additive in many processed foods. Gluten is used as a thickening agent in soups, sauces, and salad dressings. It can be added to dried spices to prevent them from clumping together. It may also be on the conveyer belt in a factory to prevent food from sticking. Gluten can be present in other surprising places such as: bouillon cubes, deli meats (bologna, sausage, hot dogs, and salami), candy (such as licorice and jelly beans), soy sauce (wheat is often the first or second ingredient), many low- or nonfat products (such as low-fat sour cream), gravy, seasonings on potato chips, imitation crabmeat, and self-basting turkeys. Even many nonfood items such as toothpaste, lipsticks, other cosmetics, and envelope glue may contain gluten. Most beers and some wine coolers contain barley malt (gluten), so they should be avoided.

Filling in The Fiber

Since the gluten-free diet eliminates many of the common grains and since most gluten-free breads and flours are low in fiber, getting enough fiber can be challenging. The American Dietetic Association (ADA) recommends a minimum of 20 to 35 grams of fiber per day, depending on calorie intake, for a healthy adult. The ADA's recommendation for children is that intake should equal age in years plus 5 grams per day (e.g. a 4-year-old should consume 9 grams per day).

Fruits, vegetables, beans, legumes, nuts, and seeds provide dietary fiber. Choose gluten-free whole grains such as wild and brown rice products over white rice products. When baking, use brown rice flour and rice bran instead of white flours. Add seeds, chopped nuts, and raisins to breads and muffins to increase the fiber in your baked goods. Amaranth, buckwheat, and millet provide 17 to 18 grams of fiber per cup. Quinoa provides 10 grams and sorghum 12 grams of fiber per cup.

If you are looking to boost your fiber intake, try adding some of these fiber-rich, gluten-free grains to your diet:

Chia is an ancient grain that produces tiny black, white, or speckled seeds, which are rich in fiber, omega-3 fatty acids, protein, calcium, magnesium, and antioxidants. One 25 gram serving (about 2 tablespoons) provides 10 grams of dietary fiber. Studies have shown that chia is low on the glycemic index, meaning that it breaks down slowly into sugar and promotes stable blood sugar levels. Chia is almost tasteless. It can be sprinkled on cereal, yogurt, and salad or baked into bread without altering the flavor.

Flaxseed is a small brown seed rich in omega-3 fatty acids, protein, fiber, vitamins, and minerals. Flaxseed has a slightly nutty flavor and, like chia, can be added to many foods and recipes. To get the benefits of the fiber and oils, look for milled flaxseed, or grind the seed yourself. The whole seeds do not break down during digestion. One serving (2 tablespoons) of milled flaxseed provides about 4 grams of fiber.

Hemp seeds are small brown seeds that contain all the essential amino acids and essential fatty acids along with various vitamins and minerals. The seeds can be eaten raw, hulled, ground into a meal, or sprouted. Hulled (shelled) hemp seeds provide about 2 grams dietary fiber per 25 gram serving. Like chia and flax, hemp can be added to cereals, yogurt, salads, and baked goods.

Psyllium husk seeds are another good source of dietary fiber. One tablespoon provides 3 grams of dietary fiber. Psyllium is used to relieve constipation, irritable bowel syndrome, diverticular disease, and diarrhea. Studies have also shown that psyllium can improve blood sugar and cholesterol levels. Psyllium seed husks are available in health food stores. Psyllium husk is also found in laxative and fiber supplements in pharmacies as granules, powders, and capsules.

Dealing With Dairy Intolerance

Milk and foods made from milk contain lactose and milk proteins (casein and whey). However, many other prepared foods can also contain these ingredients such as bread and other baked goods, processed breakfast cereals, instant potatoes, soups, breakfast drinks, margarine, lunch meats (other than kosher), salad dressings, candies and other snacks, mixes for pancakes, biscuits, and cookies, and powdered meal-replacement supplements. Even products labeled nondairy, such as powdered coffee creamer and whipped toppings, may actually include ingredients that are derived from milk and, therefore, contain lactose.

Learn to read food labels with care, looking not only for milk and lactose, but also for words such as whey, curds, milk by-products, dry milk solids, and nonfat dry milk powder. If any of these words are listed on a label, the product could contain lactose and milk proteins.

Chapter 4

Surviving And Thriving Without Gluten

Adopting a gluten-free diet will require some changes to the way you cook, shop, and dine out. For a person newly diagnosed with celiac, it can seem daunting since so many prepared foods contain gluten. But with time, you will find that the gluten-free diet is really not that difficult. And best of all, it is a healthy diet!

Shopping Gluten Free

Years ago, gluten-free products could only be found in health food stores, but now many regular grocery stores carry them. Both the selection and the availability have greatly improved over the years.

Start with your local grocery store, and see what products are safe. If you live in a small town, the selection may be more limited. However, if you speak to the store manager, he or she may be willing to special order items for you. Some of the major grocery chains now have dedicated health food sections that provide a range of gluten free products including bread, pizza, pasta, cookies, cakes, and crackers.

Gluten-free products are usually more expensive than the regular products. You can often save money by buying products by the case, shopping in bulk stores for pasta and gluten-free flours, and shopping online. If you have a favorite product, then contact the manufacturer and request coupons.

Reading Labels

It is essential to read labels, which are often imprecise, and to learn how to identify ingredients that may contain hidden gluten. As mentioned earlier, gluten can be hidden in some very surprising places. In many cases, you will not see the words "gluten" on a food label. Gluten can be present in the following ingredients: hydrolyzed vegetable or plant protein, modified food starch, textured vegetable protein, thickener, malt extract, malt flavoring, and seasonings. Check www.celiac.com or contact your local celiac association for a more complete list.

When in doubt about the ingredients or safety of a product, contact the manufacturer. Most food product labels contain a contact number or Web site for the company. Most of the larger food companies have customer relations staff ready to answer questions about their product ingredients.

Setting Up Your Gluten-Free Kitchen

Here are a few things to keep in mind when going gluten-free:

- Use a separate toaster to avoid contamination from regular breads.
- Use a separate strainer for gluten-free pasta. Even with thorough washing, strainers can retain little bits of cooked pasta that can be a problem for a celiac.
- Have a No Double-Dipping rule for butter, margarine, peanut butter, jams, and other sauces, condiments, or products in a jar. Even a few crumbs can be a problem. If this is difficult for your other family members to adhere to, then have your own separate containers marked gluten-free.
- Keep a separate cupboard for your gluten-free supplies.
- Have a supply of various gluten-free flours on hand to substitute into recipes, such as rice flour, tapioca flour, sorghum flour, potato starch, buckwheat, and xanthan gum.
- Educate your family about the gluten-free diet and how to prevent cross-contamination.

Cooking Gluten-Free

For those who are newly diagnosed with celiac, cooking gluten-free will require some experimenting and clever substitutions. Almost any recipe can be adapted to become gluten-free. Here are some tips to keep in mind for gluten-free cooking:

- Read over the recipe before you start cooking, and look up any ingredients that you are not familiar with. Remember that wheat can be under many different names such as graham and durum.
- Avoid recipes that call for premade sauces or soups since they may contain gluten. Working from scratch takes more time, but then you can be assured all ingredients are safe.
- Use cornstarch or sweet rice flour in place of regular flour to thicken sauces and gravies. Don't overheat them since starches break down and get thin when heated too long.
- Save broken pieces of bread or the end crusts of your loaf to make your own bread crumbs. Place them in a pan, air-dry for eight hours, and then grind in a food processor or blender. Ground-up rice crackers or cornmeal also work well in recipes that call for bread crumbs or coatings for meats.
- Many recipes for casseroles and stews or soups call for prepared soup broth. Either make your own and freeze it so it is handy, or keep some gluten-free bouillon cubes or broths on hand.

- Invest in some gluten-free cookbooks. There are numerous gluten-free cookbooks available created by those who have gone through the experimenting and the trial and error. For a list of suggested cookbooks and recipes, check out the Resource section in the back of this booklet.

Since it is the gluten in wheat flour that binds and gives structure to bread, baked goods, and other foods, achieving a similar consistency in gluten-free baked goods requires substituting wheat flour with a combination of gluten-free flours. Here are some of my top recommended flour blends, courtesy of cookbook author Carol Fenster:

Rice Flour Blend

3 cups brown rice flour

$1\frac{1}{4}$ cups potato starch or cornstarch

$\frac{3}{4}$ cup tapioca flour

Bean Flour Blend

2 cups potato starch or cornstarch

$1\frac{2}{3}$ cups garbanzo/fava flour

$\frac{2}{3}$ cup tapioca flour

$\frac{2}{3}$ cup sorghum flour

Sorghum Flour Blend

$1\frac{1}{2}$ cups sorghum flour

$1\frac{1}{2}$ cups potato starch

1 cup tapioca flour

$\frac{1}{2}$ cup corn flour*, chestnut flour, or bean flour

*grind white cornmeal into flour with small coffee grinder

Reprinted with permission from Carol Fenster, author of 1,000 Gluten-Free Recipes *(Wiley, 2008). www.SavoryPalate.com*

You can refrigerate or freeze these blends, but bring them to room temperature before using.

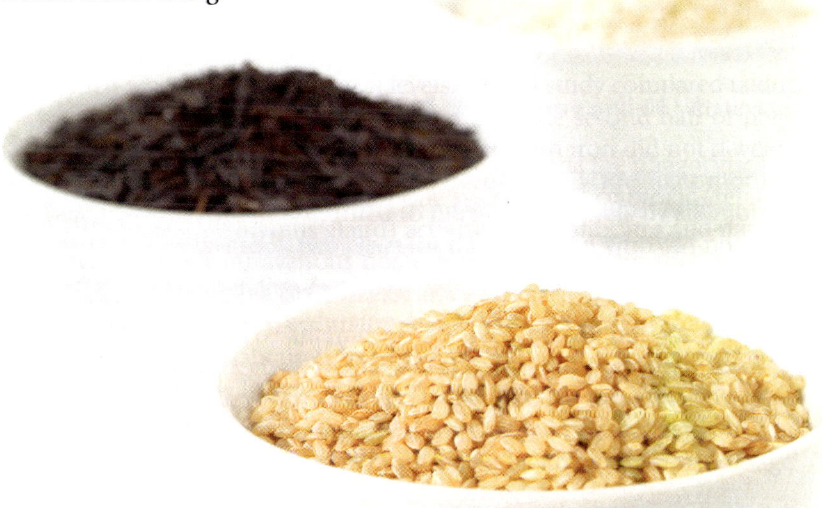

Eating Out Gluten Free

Visiting a restaurant doesn't have to be an unpleasant experience. With a little planning and some precautions, celiacs can enjoy a meal out. Before going to a particular restaurant, call ahead and ask to speak to the manager or chef to see if they can accommodate your diet. Don't assume that they will know about celiac and gluten. Take a few minutes to explain your diet. Be specific about what gluten is and the risk of cross-contamination with cutting boards and preparation bowls. Ask about marinades, sauces, and coatings on meats. See if their restaurant offers gluten-free options or if they can adapt menu items.

If you don't have the chance to call ahead, then ask to speak to the chef when you arrive. Going right to the source of the food preparation is always best since most servers will not know what gluten is and the exact ingredients in the various dishes, and the message can be lost in transit. Have a paper copy of your diet on hand that you can give to the chef. That way, he can take it to the kitchen if need be to verify any ingredients. Many celiac associations provide restaurant cards, or you can make up your own. Keep in mind that if you are special ordering a meal, it may take longer to be prepared, but it will be worth the wait.

When attending a wedding or banquet, call ahead and speak to the food and beverage manager. They appreciate knowing of your dietary needs in advance, and in my experience, most are very accommodating. Not only do they want you to enjoy your meal, but they don't want you to get sick at their function.

Even with all these precautions, cross-contamination or inadvertent exposure to gluten can occur. Refer to the next chapter of this booklet for information about a gluten digesting enzyme supplement that can help minimize the impact of hidden gluten in the diet.

Traveling Gluten Free

Taking a trip, especially to a foreign country, can be a bit daunting for a celiac since it means eating away from the comfort and safety of home and your own controls. However, a little extra planning will help to ensure a safe trip. Here are a few tips to consider:

- Contact the local tourist office in the country that you will be visiting to see if they have information on area restaurants that are celiac friendly and health food stores where you can pick up gluten-free snacks.
- Do an Internet search, and see if you can find a celiac association in the country you are visiting. They will likely be able to recommend local restaurants and stores and provide other important

information. They may also be able to provide a translation of your diet into the local language.

- When booking a flight, request a gluten-free meal. Most long-haul flights that offer a meal service will have a gluten-free option available, but they typically have to be ordered two days prior to departure. Notify the flight attendant of your diet when you are seated, so your meal doesn't inadvertently go to someone else. If the flight does not offer a meal, then eat before you get on the plane and bring snacks with you such as energy bars, crackers, nuts, seeds, and dried fruit.
- Notify the hotel of your dietary needs. Fax or e-mail a detailed description of your diet before you arrive. If they don't carry gluten-free bread or products, they may be able to order them in for you.
- Take along a gluten- and casein-digesting enzyme supplement to help ensure you are protected from hidden gluten in foods. Refer to the Resource section at the back of the booklet for information about the supplement I recommend.

When traveling to a country where English is not commonly spoken, have your dietary requirements translated into the local language. The website www.celiactravel.com provides the gluten-free diet guidelines that can be downloaded in 42 languages free of charge. You can also order cards through Triumph Dining at www.triumphdining.com

Some areas are easier to visit than others for a celiac. Traveling to Europe, especially the Scandinavian countries, is a lot easier because celiac disease is prevalent in these areas, and the hotels and restaurants are familiar with the diet. It is quite common for European restaurants to offer gluten-free menu items and even have gluten-free bread on hand. Great Britain, Australia, and New Zealand also have good awareness of celiac and the gluten-free diet. These places have good food-labeling laws that require identification of allergens such as gluten. In my experience, traveling to Asia can be more challenging since the awareness of celiac is low, there is a strong language barrier, and many of the foods are prepared with wheat-containing soy sauce.

Gluten in Drugs And Supplements

Although people with celiac disease are cautious about what they eat, it is also important to realize that gluten can be found in medications as well as vitamin and herbal supplements. Gluten is added to medications as an excipient, which binds the ingredients in the pill together. There are several types of excipients that drug companies use, including corn and wheat, so it is important always to check with your pharmacist. When in doubt, contact the manufacturer to find out if the particular medication you are taking is gluten-free.

Chapter 5
Supplemental Support

Nutritional supplements can play an important role in optimizing health. Prior to starting the gluten-free diet, many celiacs go years without diagnosis. The intestinal damage caused by years of ingesting gluten can be significant. Since nutrient absorption occurs through the intestine, undiagnosed celiac can result in malnutrition and signs of nutrient deficiency such as anemia, skin rash, fatigue, poor cognitive function, and stunted growth of hair and nails. Additionally, the gluten-free diet, while healthy, can be lacking in certain nutrients. Gluten free flours are lower in fiber and not enriched with iron and B vitamins.

Supplements can help facilitate healing of the body, aid digestion, and compensate for possible dietary deficiencies. Below are some supplements celiacs may want to consider:

Multivitamin And Mineral Complex

Fruits and vegetables provide us with our primary sources of vitamins and minerals. However, the nutrient levels of our produce has greatly declined over the past few decades. Fruits and vegetables are grown in nutrient-depleted soil, picked before they are ripe, and sprayed with pesticides. All these factors decrease nutrient levels.

There are many factors that deplete nutrients in our body and increase our need for vitamins and minerals. These factors include stress, smoking, and the use of prescription drugs (such as diuretics, birth control pills, blood pressure medications, and cholesterol-lowering drugs). As noted above, celiacs have increased needs because of malabsorption and the fact that many gluten-free products do not contain the same level of nutrients as regular products.

The purpose of a multivitamin is to ensure that your body is getting all essential nutrients required for good health. Look for a product in capsule or liquid form, which is easier to digest. Hard-coated tablets may have coatings and dyes that impair absorption. Of course, it is also important to make sure that your vitamin and all other supplements you take are gluten-free. Some companies add gluten as a binder. Note: Those with iron-deficiency anemia may need more iron than a multivitamin provides. Check with your health care provider.

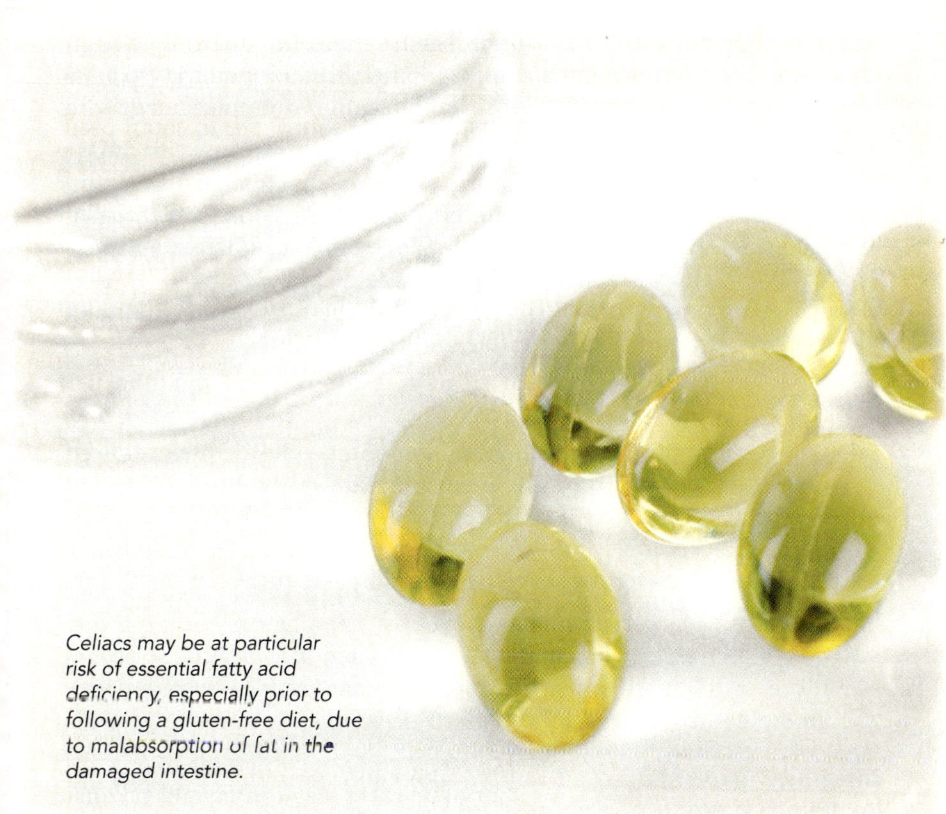

Celiacs may be at particular risk of essential fatty acid deficiency, especially prior to following a gluten-free diet, due to malabsorption of fat in the damaged intestine.

Essential Fatty Acids (EFAs)

EFAs are good fats that are essential for health throughout life. They are required for growth and development of the brain, nervous system, adrenal glands, sex organs, and eyes. They maintain the health of cell membranes, produce hormones and brain chemicals, and regulate various cell processes.

The body cannot make EFAs, so they must be obtained through diet or supplementation. The two main classes of EFAs are the omega-3s and omega-6s. Celiacs may be at particular risk of essential fatty acid deficiency, especially prior to following a gluten-free diet, due to malabsorption of fat in the damaged intestine.

Omega-6s are found abundantly in vegetable and seed oils. Omega-3s are present in fish and, to a lesser extent, in some plants (chia seed, flaxseed, and leafy green vegetables). Omega-3 deficiency is thought to be quite common, and supplementing with omega-3s has been shown to offer a number of health benefits, such as reducing the risk of heart attack and improving brain function and skin health. Omega-3 supplements are also recommended for women trying to get pregnant or who are pregnant since these good fats are essential to the growing brain, eyes, and nervous system of the baby.

Fish oil provides the highest amount of omega-3s. Look for a pharmaceutical grade, cold-pressed fish oil from a reputable manufacturer. Those who cannot tolerate fish oils can take chia seed oil or flaxseed oil. The usually dosage for omega-3s is 1 to 3 grams daily. There are specific formulas for children with improved taste and texture.

Digestive Enzymes

Digestive enzymes are found naturally in raw foods and are produced to some extent by the body. These enzymes aid in the breakdown and digestion of food and may be particularly beneficial to those with celiac, who face impaired digestion and nutrient absorption. There are three classes: Proteolytic enzymes digest protein, lipases digest fat, and amylases digest carbohydrates.

A new digestive enzyme supplement designed specifically for celiacs and those with gluten and casein sensitivity has recently become available in the United States and Canada. This supplement provides a wide range of plant enzymes to support complete digestion of all types of nutrients, such as carbohydrates, proteins, and fats, with targeted support for the digestion of gluten and casein. Our ability to produce these enzymes declines as we age, which can contribute to gluten and casein sensitivity.

This supplement is unique because it is active across a broad pH range in the digestive tract and it contains a specific enzyme called DPP IV, which has been shown to aid in the breakdown of gluten and gliadin from foods. This product is intended to support the gluten-free and casein-free diet. Celiacs and those with casein sensitivity must always be very strict in avoiding gluten and casein at all times. Yet, despite one's best efforts to avoid gluten and casein, there are so many hidden sources. Plus, contamination may occur when eating at restaurants. Taking specific enzymes before risky meals will aid digestion and help to defend against hidden gluten and casein. For more information refer to the resource section in the back of this booklet.

Probiotics

Also known as friendly or beneficial bacteria, probiotics, such as acidophilus, are normally present in the mouth, digestive and urinary tracts, and vaginal area. Probiotics provide many health benefits: They protect against infection from harmful bacteria (yeast and bacteria); aid in detoxification; produce B vitamins; aid digestion; and support immune function. They can improve bowel function and aid both constipation and diarrhea. Celiacs may be deficient in probiotics because of intestinal damage.

Probiotics are present in some fermented dairy foods (live culture yogurt), although the potency and stability is questionable. Look for a quality probiotic supplement that is designed to survive stomach acid, which can deliver the beneficial bacteria to the intestine. Also ensure that the product is stable at room temperature, so no refrigeration is required.

There are other supplements that may be necessary depending on one's individual health status. For example, celiacs are at risk of osteoporosis and may require additional bone-building nutrients such as calcium, magnesium, and vitamin D. Those with diabetes, thyroid disease, or other issues may require other supplements. It is important to consult with your health care provider if you have any health concerns and before you start taking any new drugs or supplements.

Summary

For those who have struggled with horrible symptoms for years, having a diagnosis of celiac disease can be a sigh of relief. Unlike many chronic conditions, most celiacs do not require medications. The disease can be managed effectively with a gluten-free diet, and supplements can play a supportive role in restoring and optimizing health.

Becoming gluten-free is easier today than ever before. There is growing awareness of celiac disease among practitioners. Food manufacturers and restaurants recognize the importance of serving the growing number of people who are gluten intolerant, so we are likely to see major advances in the availability and variety of gluten-free products in years to come.

The move to gluten-free living can bring about a number of positive life changes. Reading labels makes you an informed consumer; the gluten-free diet is a healthy diet since it encourages fresh, unprocessed foods; and going gluten-free can dramatically improve your health and well-being.

Resources

Books And Magazines

Beyond Rice Cakes: A Young Person's Guide to Cooking, Eating & Living Gluten-Free by Vanessa Maltin This book offers hilarious stories about living with celiac, as well as recipes, cooking tips, and advice from experts.

Celiac Disease, a Hidden Epidemic by Peter H. R. Green and Rory Jones This book explains how celiac disease is properly diagnosed, treated, and managed.

Complete Gluten-Free Cookbook by Donna Washburn and Heather Butt This book provides 150 gluten-free, lactose-free recipes, many with egg-free variations, as well as nutritional analyses.

Gluten-Free Cooking for Dummies by Danna Korn and Connie Sarros This book has information covering food preparation, purchasing gluten-free products and ingredients, saving money, and nutritional value of foods.

Gluten-Free Diet by Shelley Case, RD This book provides detailed food and ingredient information and a directory of gluten-free product manufacturers, bakeries, and stores.

Gluten-Free Living This quarterly magazine is devoted to gluten-free living, with articles on eating and cooking gluten-free and reading labels.

Living Without This magazine provides information and recipes for those with food allergies and sensitivities.

Waiter, Is There Wheat in My Soup? The Official Guide on Dining Out, Shopping, and Traveling Gluten-Free and Allergen-Free by LynnRae Ries This book provides information on dining out, shopping gluten-free, and advice from chefs, national support groups, and those living gluten-free.

1,000 Gluten-Free Recipes by Carol Fenster, PhD This book is loaded with tasty gluten-free recipes, tips on baking, shopping guidelines, pointers on reading food labels, and more. She is the author of several other cookbooks.

Food And Supplement Manufacturers

There are many excellent gluten-free manufacturers. Here are some of my favorites:

Bob's Red Mill (www.bobsredmill.com) produces a full line of certified gluten-free products, including flours and baking mixes.

El Peto (www.elpeto.com) offers a range of breads, bagels, muffins, pies, cookies, pastas, baking mixes, and pizza crusts.

Enjoy Life Foods (www.enjoylifefoods.com) offers cereals, bagels, cookies, granola and snack bars that are free of the 8 most common allergens, including gluten and dairy.

Enzymatic Therapy (www.enzy.com) offers high-quality dietary supplements, including gluten-digesting enzymes, probiotics and fish oils, available at health food stores throughout North America.

Glutino (www.glutino.com) offers a range of breads, bagels, muffins, cupcakes, pretzels, baking mixes, pizza crusts, and frozen dinners.

Kinnikinnick (www.kinnikinnick.com Kinnikinnick offers a range of breads, bagels, muffins, donuts, cookies, bars, pretzels, baking mixes, and pizza crusts.

LARABAR (www.larabar.com) offers a wide range of snack bars made of unsweetened fruits, nuts, and spices. They are free of gluten, dairy, and soy, made from 100 percent whole food, and are vegan, high in fiber, and available in many tasty flavors.

Nature's Path (www.naturespath.com) offers a range of delicious cereals, snack bars, and waffles.

Pamela's Products (www.pamelasproducts.com) offers a range of cookies, biscotti, and baking mixes for bread, pizza, and cakes.

Pure Bar (www.thepurebar.com) Pure Bars are USDA certified organic, raw, gluten-free, high-fiber, vegan, Kosher, and best of all they taste great. Made with fruit and nuts (no added sugar), they are amazingly chewy and sweet.

Web sites

BioCard Celiac Test www.celiachometest.com This home-test kit for celiac disease is as accurate as laboratory blood screening and is available without a prescription.

Canadian Celiac Association www.celiac.ca *Mission:* The Canadian Celiac Association is a national organization dedicated to providing services and support to persons with celiac disease and dermatitis herpetiformis through programs of awareness, advocacy, education, and research.

Celiac Disease Foundation www.celiac.org *Mission:* To develop awareness and improve the quality of medical and self-care for celiac disease/dermatitis herpetiformis; and to provide telephone information and referral services, free information, a medical advisory board, and special educational seminars and general meetings.

Celiac Sprue Association www.csaceliacs.org *Mission:* To provide information and educational materials for persons with celiac sprue and dermatitis herpetiformis and for parents of children with celiac disease. CSA is made up of six regions, with chapters and resource units across the US.

Celiac Travel (www.celiactravel.com) provides facts, tips, and tales to help maintain your special diet anywhere in the world. They offer (free) gluten-free restaurant cards in 42 languages. They also have a blog with daily gluten-free recipes.

Celiac.com (www.celiac.com) was founded in 1995 by Scott Adams, a person with celiac whose goal is "To help as many people as possible with celiac disease get diagnosed and live a happy, healthy, gluten-free life." Adams provides a wealth of information about celiac disease, diagnosis, treatment, recipes, product information, research initiatives, and more.

Gluten-Free MD (www.glutenfreemd.com) provides educational products for health care professionals and those with celiac disease.

Gluten Intolerance Group of North America (GIG) www.gluten.net *Mission:* to increase awareness by providing accurate, up-to-date information, education, and support to those with gluten intolerance, celiac disease/dermatitis herpetiformis, their families, health care professionals, and the general public.

National Celiac Foundation www.celiaccentral.org NFCA is a non-profit organization dedicated to raising awareness and funding for celiac disease that will advance research, education and screening amongst medical professionals, children and adults.

Savory Palate www.savorypalate.com Carol Fenster, PhD, offers a variety of outstanding, gluten-free/allergen-free cookbooks, as well as information and resources on celiac disease.

Selected References

Bardella MT, Elli L, Velio P, et al. Silent celiac disease is frequent in the siblings of newly diagnosed celiac patients. *Digestion* 75:182-187, 2007.

Catassi C, Fabiani E, Rätsch IM, et al. The coeliac iceberg in Italy. A multicentre antigliadin antibodies screening for coeliac disease in school-age subjects. *Acta Paediatrica* 85:29-35, 1996.

Eaton W, Morensen PB, Agerbo E, et al. Coeliac disease and schizophrenia: population based case control study with linkage of Danish national registers. *BMJ* 328:438-9, 2004.

Fasano A, Berti I, Gerarduzzi T, et al. Prevalence of celiac disease in at-risk and not-at-risk groups in the United States. *Arch Intern Med* 163:286-92, 2003.

Fassano A and Catassi C. Current approaches to diagnosis and treatment of celiac disease: an evolving spectrum. *Gastroenterology* 120:636-51, 2001.

Goggins M and Kelleher D. Celiac disease and other nutrient related injuries to the gastrointestinal tract. *The American Journal of Gastroenterology* 89(8):S2-S17, 1994.

Green PH, et al. Characteristics of Adult Celiac Disease in the USA: Results of a Nation Survey. *American Journal of Gastroenterology*, 2001.

Halsted CH. The many faces of celiac disease. *N Engl J Med* 334(18):1190-1, 1996.

Holmes, GK, Prior, P, Lane, MR, et al. Malignancy in coeliac disease—effect of a gluten free diet. *Gut* 30:333-8; doi:10.1136/gut.30.3.333, 1989.

Johnstone DE and Roghmann KJ. Recommendations for soy infant formula: a review of the literature and a survey of pediatric allergists. *Pediatr Asthma Allergy Immunol* 7:77-88, 1993.

Meloni GF, Dessole S, Vargiu N, et a.. The prevalence of celiac disease in infertility. *Human Reproduction* 14(11):2759-61, 1999.

Rewers M. Epidemiology of celiac disease: What are the prevalence, incidence, and progression of celiac disease? *Gastroenterology*. 128(4):S47-S51, 2005.

West J. Celiac disease and its complications: a time traveller's perspective. *Gastroenterology* 136(1):32-4, 20006.

For more information about the author of this booklet visit

www.sherrytorkos.com